2016

Author. Jay Kay

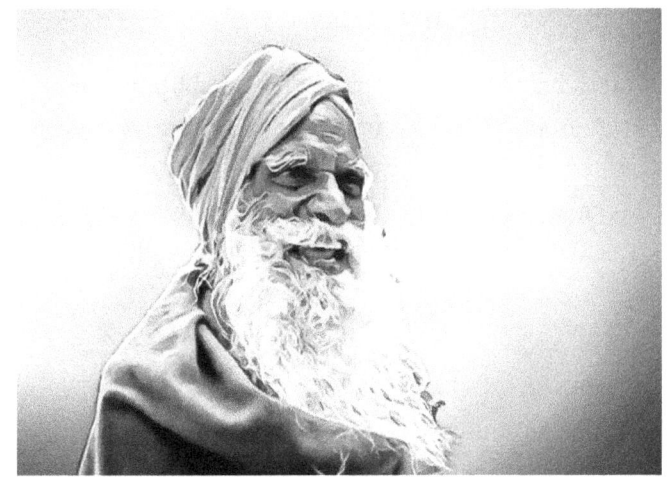

Messiah of Organic Farming – G. Nammalvar

From InOrganic to ORGANIC!

This book is intended to create an awareness campaign of looming DEATH to LIFE, in order to revive LIFE with importance of Organic food. It is a campaign against the odds; those who destroy NATURE in the name of rapid Industrialization with excerpts of Dr. G.Namalvar's, Agriculture pledge to save Nature & human beings. It is a quest for survival!!!

© Jay Kay 2016.

Published by
Jay Kay
writerjaykay@gmail.com

To my Gurus, Maharishi Vethathiri & the Buddha, G. Namazhvar, messiah of Organic farming who is a Divine Guru for all farmers across the world and environmentalists. The contemporary leader Piyush Manush, India who inspired me by developing forests. I would like to thank Sir Albert Howard was a British botanist for his contributions to the Indian agriculturist.

Finally, my family, friends & publishers with gratitude… and above all my Divine Nature throbbing in me!

Thank you for all your patience and guidance…

<u>Organic</u>!

Oh Nature-Organic is your Nature!
Humans are In-Organic,
They extract everything from you;
And destroy you!

Oh Nature,
I see you cry,
For all that humans have done!
In the name of Industry!

I seek amnesty for all humans,
From Nature to animals!
For all barbaric things
That humans have done till date!

A messiah has arrived,
G. Nummular, the savior
To arise, awake and STOPNOT
Till the World is saved from
The perils of extinction!
Save Thy Nature!!!

- Jay kay

PREFACE

The human consciousness has evolved to the extent that it can understand its inherent nature in scientific inquiry. Perhaps, you can realize it through self-realization with the determined practices of yoga and meditation. It is time to realize that each of you're part of the ultimate Nature by revelations of truth. You must stop abusing Nature or else you'd eventually face the brink of human extinction. Predominantly, the West is outward bound, whilst East is inward bound, where there had been several revelations of truth by several enlightened masters from time-to-time. The western countries have introduced chemical fertilizers such as ammonia used during the world war. These products such as potassium, ammonia, naptha, sulphate with UREA chemical fertilizers are poisoning soil and essentially your blood. This is the one of the root causes of cancer. While you're aware of healthy exercise, you're not even aware of the poison that you're consumer on a daily basis. In the name of 'Green Revolution', countries like South America used chemical fertilizers to increase the yield/hectare.

G. Nammalvar is one of the few and rarest of the world community, who had served relentlessly for the welfare of the organic Agri-culture all over the world. It is a culture of cultivating food for all and it is considered as divine in India unlike the western culture claiming it to be Agri business. The moment business got in to the fields of producing food; it has violated the basic integrity of producing chemical free food to all citizens of the World. Instead, these companies producing food, use various types of chemical fertilizers used as pesticide, herbicide resulting in genocide. It is time for a revolution as government seems to be interested in political interests alone without considering welfare of the people.

Reference:
https://www.youtube.com/watch?v=R1AUcR_HwhM

I'd like to start by saluting these great men of the centuries. Maharishi Vethathiri, who tirelessly contributed to one world governance to support a sustainable living in unison with Nature? One of his key notes to the UNO was very effective focused on one global nation. Needless to state, World has converged in to one from any products that you use in a daily life. However, with this rapid globalization the arrival of diseases had been globalized too. Perhaps there is strong need to change the judiciary, legislature and executive system all over the world. For better governance, it is essential to start from the scratch by creating a proper government.

Perhaps a real democracy is required for the people, by the PEOPLE of the World without any geographical barriers. A lot of consolidation is required to eliminate old ways of thinking in the west to inculcate best practices that has real values in life. The purpose of western life should change from outward bound to inward realizing the values of life. This is only possible by inculcating virtues in life in every individual through meditation which should become way of life as visualized by Maharishi Vethathiri by living in unison with Nature and not by challenging Nature.

From time memorial, Indian ecologists have contributed to the society by harnessing the power of Nature. It is very simple as they taught people to live in unison and allow nature to do it including healing best practices such as Ayurveda, siddha and unani. They had taught people to worship Nature as God. Hence, most of these facts of living in unison had always been part of the Indian culture. However, In the name of rapid industrialization, greedy politicians seem to be threating the citizens with chemicals everywhere, thus polluting Mother Nature.

I would like to introduce you to messiah of the Organic farming, G. Nammalvar. A lot of farmers were trapped into debts in India, who were unable to repay and committed suicide. One of the reasons of poor yield is due to rapid usage of chemical fertilizers with cost of production due to low yield/hectare. Further, Indian farmers struggled to repay huge loans due to the banks for procuring chemical fertilizers, which has almost deteriorated soil. Thus, farmers have lost the soil with huge debts to repay. Similar debts mounted in farmers using genetically modified seeds from a corporate called 'MONSON-TO'. They had to repay a % profit on the yield for using these seeds. What a pity? How can a government allow corporates to impose such a rule? It is like imperialistic approach.

Our legendary agriculturist, G. Nammalvar spent his whole life for the welfare of the agricultural farmer communities all over the World to spread about conservation and importance of organic farming. G. Nammalvar is the one among legends who helped many farmers in India and the World.

I feel the real problem is lack of universal thinking aligned with Nature. It's time to think universally in sync with the Nature, meaning industries that do not harm Nature and agriculture that is sustainable without any usage of fertilizers that are poisonous. Each of should rise up and condemn any technology that harms Nature.

The objectives of this book are to help you understand the perils of food produced by the major corporate agriculture and the practices of using chemical fertilizers such as DIOXIN that your children consume every day. With Bio-Technology (BT) seeds modified using genetic engineering is causing more harm to the human body. Further, BT-Brinjal, BT-potato will cause cancer, hence citizens of the world should stop this coming to the consumer market. These fertilizers eventually cause CANCER. Also, enlighten you about broader views of Corporate America with rapid industrialization that is poisoning Mother Earth. I urge people of America to rise up and stop production of chemical fertilizers.

For heaven's sake, do not export into other countries, as India has already started the Monsanto production in Telangana and Gujarat. As you know, prevention is better than cure. At least you can form social forms to create awareness campaigns in respective part of the world. Eventually, Nature will help you in the campaign to alleviate from the sufferings. I strongly feel a Swadesh movement is required to stop such barbaric activities into our culture.

I'd like to invoke blessings of my beloved spiritual Guru, Maharishi Vethathiri and the Buddha. Foremost, the spirit of the Organic messiah, G. Nammalvar, who tirelessly worked throughout his life for the welfare of the society. He has created awareness about the Organic farming in every nook and corner of the World. I would like to invoke his soul to guide me to share his visions and solution for all impending problems of the World. Indeed, each of the factors contributes to the global warming.

I would like to request every citizen of the World to realize the looming threats to Nature and your health due to greedy politicians those who have commercialized and poisoned food. I would like you to insist 'FDA' in the United States to pass food bills to protect the World citizens. US has done the damage with consequences of mass destruction to the world citizens, hence I would like to pledge to the US government to save the World. Beware of consuming poison in daily food that you eat. It's time to raise awareness and start protesting as one world citizen to unite the world. East or West is just boundary created by human minds. It is all one and the same as Maharishi Vethathiri mentioned. He stated in Nature there is nothing called as deficit as she ever loves.

Only the human minds are greedy due to lack of realization of truth.

***

Chapter 1

Organic vs. Inorganic!

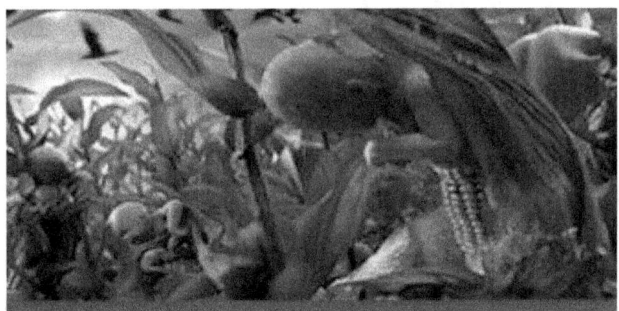

"We now live in a nation where
doctors destroy health, lawyers destroy
justice, universities destroy knowledge,
governments destroy freedom,
the press destroys information,
religion destroys morals, and our banks
destroy the economy." ~ Chris Hedges 6
Source: OrganicLiveFood

Today as we speak, World has many problems with looming threats of food poisoning with the above witnessing statement of Christ Hedges. Today, we are in a world where a doctor prescribes medicines for his wellness and a lawyer extends the case eternally. All morals in life seems to be violated in earning wealth at any cost, without realizing the impact that is causing in the society.

What you sow is what you'd eventually get? Isn't so? If you're a renowed Industrialist amassing wealth at the expense of others, how would you expect your own family to lead a happy life. It's a simple law of Nature. If you're working against Nature, then obviously the results would be wrong. A simple example of alchohol consumption, smoking cigarates would result in cancer. Now, if you're further involved in immoral activities, your health will be spoiled. What is the purpose of life ?

There is a growing trend of generation x indulging in mundane pleasures without even realizing the long-term harmful effects. How would you react, if you're diagnosed with cancer! God willing 'no'! But, my point is that you should refrain from activities that would cause harm to self, society and Nature. Everyone would concur if I say 'Nature is God' and the same mass is within you.

You're part of the Divine Nature, hence there is no need to work against it. Why the hell are you cutting trees and killing forests which is resulting in a major ecological diaster? What non-sense is this! You're investing in forecasting global warming, venture in the mars and moon! Can't Government take steps to avert a major diaster using law to protect Nature and use law and enforcement to avoid chemicals used in fertilizers. It's all due to greedy politicians all over the world, indulging in amassing wealth.

These chemical fertilizers originated from world war (I) and (II) where it was used for bio-weapons of mass destructions. Now, these factories are using it as chemical fertilizers to kill soil wealth to remain profitable. It's a mer business strategy. Moreso, your blood has been poisoned. Then , the result would be diseases in the body! This is what is happening with the reducing life-span of human beings, animals and Nature itself with a major ecological diaster in the pipeline. Further, you're foolishly giving profit to the greedy politicians by consuming alchohol as a consumer.

Indeed, first time in the evolution of human beings there is a trend of parents in mid-forties seeing their children growing obese. You're slowly poisoning children. How would you expect a long life-span of your children, if you're not even aware of the slow poison in food. Why can't you insist respective governments to use science and technology to harness Nature. A simple mobile 'app'can predict analytics of how much chemical fertilizer has been mixed in produce. The same applies in industrialization of Agriculture by using traditional methods of farming combined with modern equipments. However, you should be cognizant of not eating away farmer's profit by rapid industrialization. It should be carefully industrialized by involving all these farming using co-operative farming by leveraging indigenous techniques.

I feel there is a lack of holistic approach in the world today. A lack of complete thinking from modern medicines to food. I am allopathy is good for surgery, but not for treating diabetes, cancer or any other diseases. It is staggering to hear that there is no treatment for cancer, then why the hell are these so called doctors booking profit in the name of treatment. A holistic approach is required by combining homeopathy, siddha and ayurvedic medicines with allopathy. You've been abusing body with the usage of allopathy medicines and same is true with the usage of chemical fertilizers, both your body and Nature are equally abused.

Perhaps, you're not leaving a planet for the future generations to come. The ultimate purpose of life is to live in unison with Nature, enjoy all wealth and move on without abusing it. But, your minds have become greedy in the name of wealth, gold etc. hence, mostly western world has industrialized everything with chemicals to gain more and more for themselves. Further, these exports to the developing countries have killed all indigenous ways of farming in South America, India and rest of the World.

I believe countries like United States can gain tremendous insights from ancient Indian farm techniques. Dr. Nammalvar has introduced simple and natural farm methods to empower poor farmers. Why can't we support them if not abuse them! The food that you eat is in the hands of poor farmers, then why don't we escalate this matter to the governments in the respective countries to peacefully protest against inorganic methods involving usage of plastics, chemicals usage etc.

One of the visions of Maharishi Vethathiri was '**One Governance**' as basic human needs are same for everyone in the world. Indeed, Mararishi has requested UNO to discuss long term strategies of communalizing boundaries of every country under one leadership of UNO. This would completely stop wars/conflict between countries, resulting in huge savings to every government, which could be utilized for scientific and natural ways of farming. It is possible only by the power of every individual forming an ocean of bliss against the odds of the illicit governance. To extend his philosophy, I'd say we can globalize money across the world with single currency. Also, it is possible to globalize food production to support farmers worldwide and stop any chemical usage.

It is important to understand why Indian farmers have lost production resulted in many suicides in the last decade. A country that had immense wealth to feed the whole world is struggling to revive its own farming. Did you analyze the reason? It is simple. India followed the techniques of Western world in trying to mimic their process of increasing yield / hectare by using chemical fertilizers such as pesticides. This usage had resulted in killing the soil wealth and further damaged the ecology by killing all good insects around such as bee's and micro-organisms under the soil. A consistent usage of chemical fertilizers has resulted in low yield, which caused farmers to increase the usage of chemicals more and more. Finally, soil has lost its wealth, food has been poisoned. Further, farmers couldn't repay the loans provided by the respective banks. What is staggering is that government of India has not taken enough steps to stop these chemical fertilizers and its usage in the Indian soil. My wish is that as citizens of the world, you should raise awareness and insist governments to invest in agriculture using indigenous techniques all over the world. As stated by Dr. G. Nammalvar, soil can be revived using:

    a.   Soil should be soft. This can be done by using cow dung.
    b.   Bacteria, colon, worms should be availabe in the soil. This would result in organic wealth (magnesium, iron)

The United states of America said these above techniques were ancient. By using computer technology and yield/hectare calculations, they have brain washed all farmers in India to use modern techniques with the usage of chemical fertilizers. All these BT (bio-technology) is not good. All science seems to be foolish to kill Nature and humans. This is reason for cancer and reducing life span in India and rest of the world. G. Namalvar goes a step further stating that we have lost the wealth of soil in India by using chemical fertilizers. The usage of cattle has been lost. The Indian scientists have not used any research to understand the impact of the above diaster. In those days, magnesium consumed by cows came out of calcium in milk. It was a natural process. Now, the scientists have messed up using modern techniques in the name of science.

The usage of our ancient organic fertilizers such as 'Panchagavya' can revive the soil. It is possible with each of you to support farmers. My pledge is to support farmers to avoid a major disaster. These Indian scientists have not used any intelligence to analyze the above ecological disasters. You should understand the cultural heritage of India and its farming techniques. India can produce food for the entire world. These so called scientists in the United States have caused a major disaster in the Indian farming by introducing chemical fertilizers. There is no need for these chemicals usage for increasing production. In Wayanad, Kerala, there had been a huge loss by losing soil wealth. In last decade in Kerala, TamilNadu, Karnataka and rest of India there had been reports of several farmers committed suicide. This is a staggering news and we should wake up to the situation.

As G. Namalavar said: The entire world can be saved by using natural methods for farming. His vision was not just producing yield/hectare. Indeed, his vision extends beyond farming by restoring Nature at its best. For example, use neem trees, create a biodiversity, cattle feed. There is no need for using tractors, instead use earth worms. A food chain should be developed by using natural process of transformation as illustrated in the food chain process below:

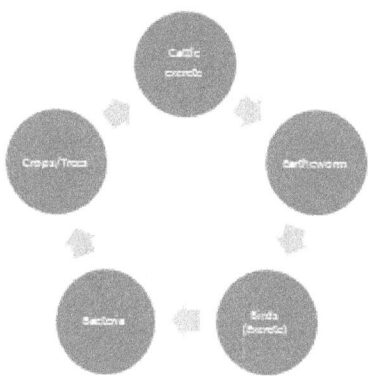

Food Chain process

In the above food chain, cattle excrete serves as food for earthworms, which in turn softens soil. In next step, birds feed these earthworms and these birds excrete feed bacteria. Thus resulting in good bacteria increasing in soil. These micro-organisms help in growing forests, crops, trees, plants etc. This is a complete bio-diversity. All these scientists seem to have convoluted thoughts in theoritical knowledge. More and more you use chemical fertilizers, all good insects have ruthlessly killed good insects, bacteria. These pesticides have killed good insects and the ecology. If a cow grazes on grass with pesticides, its milk is poisoned and naturally human beings are poisoned too by consuming milk. Dr. G. Nammalvar found a simple natural way of organic pesticide that can be prepared using cow urine such as Panchagavya etc.

Moreso, threat is that it is even more painful to hear that parents in sixties will see their children diseased. It struck my soul in past couple of weeks, when I heard about the looming threats of food poisoning due to greedy politicians all over the World. In my view, anything that you do against Nature is Inorganic. 'Organic' is living in unison with Nature through body, mind and soul. For example, I would say a thought that is not aligned with Nature is also Inorganic. Anything that you'd do against the laws of Nature is inorganic.

The Hindustan known as India had been continuously ruled by the invaders of Afghan by the Mughals in 15th century. Further, British Raj arrived at the stores of Hindustan as East India Company for trade and commerce. It started trading and then slowly colonized India for almost couple of centuries in 16th and 17th where there had been a huge influence of the western culture and industrialization imposed in the India. Hence, India had almost lost her heritage and cultural richness of the ancient times. One good thing despite all issues in the World is that the problems are also globalized. It is imperative to think alike and derive solutions for all problems globally.

Reference - Monsanto was able to manufacture 72 million liters of dioxin that was dumped and sprayed on more than 4.8 million Vietnamese civilians during the Vietnam War. As a result of Agent Orange, more than 400,000 Vietnamese died or suffered from disabilities and more than half a million children were left with birth defects. Ironically, despite all the evidences about dioxin toxicity, up to this day Monsanto claims that dioxin is not toxic and should not be banned. Please refer below for more details:

http://www.seattleorganicrestaurants.com/vegan-whole-food/Monsanto-corruption-gmo.php#sthash.qwqCOANr.dpuf

The same company has started its operations in India too...In the name of sustainable agriculture they are killing every Indian citizen those who consume these produce as it contains Dioxin which is very dangerous to our human body. It is a toxic waste and very poisonous causing CANCER.

Refer to the link below:
http://www.monsanto.com/global/in/whoweare/pages/monsanto-india-limited.aspx

What you see is what you'd perceive. As the sayings goes; *'All that glitters is not gold'. All that looks good in the United States isn't necessarily good. From packaged food, KFC, Burger King, Pizza, Coke, Pepsi, Colgate, Malt soft drinks, chocolate drinks, packaged Tuna is all contaminated.* Remember your Bollywood honchos and famous sports person endorsing these products in India is beyond comprehension. One of the senior actor had to remove portion of large intestine in India, result was due to excessive coke. He stopped all endorsing all carbonated drinks. There is a saying, *'You'd know the real pain; only if you have it'*;

Today, most of the oceans have been polluted, leaving no mercy of humans to the water world creatures. The chances of cancer are doubled by the consumption of red meat, sea food with its packaged contaminated food. It is imperative for the world citizen to become a vegan immediately to save self and Nature. This helps in reducing carbon footprint. You cannot kill poultry, cattle for food. What is the point in leading a life with diseases?

Don't you think you that should contribute to the society positively? It is important to lead a balanced life with proper yoga, meditation to keep your body, mind healthy. Therefore, you should spend time with Nature. My joy bound no limits when I planted trees as part of Elfun activities in the suburbs of Hyderabad. And my quest is increasing to live in unison with Nature. A simple life with Nature is all good enough. Believe me there is no point in amassing wealth at the expense of your health and without giving back to the society. There is nothing wrong in spending time at work, but not always without enough workouts. You should view life with a 360 degree of self, family, social and environment.

A good exercise regime to follow with a social group of like-minded people in supporting a cause such as helping poor societies or grow trees and forests like the legendary environmentalist, Piyush Manush, who is a young activist in suburbs of Salem, Tamil Nadu, India. You should live for a cause to keep yourself motivated and charged towards protecting Nature. Trust-me, Nature will heal you if you're motivated to support Nature and citizens of the world. You can adopt a village or a lake and take care of it or a school. Anything is good.

Furthermore, chemical fertilizers used as herbicide is contaminating crops at its roots, hence it is like a slow poison. All of the above factors result in causing cancer. You don't have any clew as a consumer what you're imposed to. Your body has become extremely toxic. Now, they are facing the aftermath of these inordinate desires to commercialize everything, thus resulting in various forms of diseases. The west has not even left Cancer. It has been commercialized by doctors. If you visit a hospital for curing cancer. They have commercialized diseases by creating drugs that is not doing its job! Indeed it makes your body as inorganic and doesn't allow nature healing it.

It's like the rapid industrialization has proved to be disastrous to the ecology in the outer environment, with the body, mind polluted in respective terms by chemical food. Finally, west has not even spared minds with the free flow of content in the internet showcasing women in the poorest plight as a sexual entity. Thus, the west has commoditized basic needs of food, rest, sex and work. Each of these factors has been commercialized. For example, variety of food for taste has been distributed in the restaurants and sex is commercialized too. Further, work has been made complex with time pressure to make each of you lead a stressful life. Finally, health care is a fantasy by creating so much of fear in mind and finally abusing people in the name of cancer.

Indeed, most of these diseases can be healed by Natural methods. That's it, you'd be asked for the insurance card and rest will be history until they steal all your wealth of life-time. It is apparent that most of you're consuming food that is poisonous. For all those IT engineers, doctors and nurses who flock the land of America must read the astonishing artifacts of background story to the chemical fertilizers produced in the land of America. Moreover the toxic 'dioxin' has been used in the Vietnam War with a mass genocide of 400,000 civilians.

You've to realize and be sensitive to the society and world around to be able to safeguard it, as you may not be aware of many things happening around you as often the corporates decide and you follow blindly. You'd not be aware of the real motive behind the greedy politicians and businessmen around.

World has realized the perils of Inoragnic content in food, beyond which a deep realization is required on how it impacts mind and the Universe. There is no problem in Nature, It is all created by the human mind. Nature is ever loving and it will procreate with every single seed that you sow. It will create forests if you let it grow. Human minds seems to greedy for amassing wealth. I feel more you're educated, more your head gets heavier.

The corporate goals of balance sheet is the reason for all chaos. Ironically the Agri-Culture is considered a noble job to cultivate food for human beings has been caught up in to perils of corproate America. It has done it with the support of greedy politicians and business men counting dollar bills.

This concept of mass production and gross profit is resulting in a major ecological disaster with chemical fertilizers used extensive with its waste mixed in rivers. The entire fauna and flora is slowly wiped from the World map. Now, Nature is in need of your support to protect her. It's like a mom asking for help to save her and yourself and the future generations to come. What kind of planet that you're leaving today to help your children survive in the future. You cannot make another Earth, then how can you spoil its wealth.

One side chemical fertilizers has set up a huge ecological disaster and the other side lakes are being occupied by the builders for construction of multi-storeyed buildings in the name of rapid urbanization. I fear if this trend grows, there won't be a planet Earth in the next 100 years. Hence, it is essential to think about Global Warming and actions that we need to take right now to stop these barbaric acts against Nature. It is a crime that we should stop. You can grow trees, plants and contribute in helping bio-diversity. Insist your governments to find alternative fuel, instead of petrol. Also, there are ways to produce sustainable energy instead of relying in nuclear energy. The most weakest link in India is Agriculture. If this sector flourishes then the whole World can be fed by India alone with best practices followed simply organic.

Nature has gracefully evoved with a beautiful mind to live in unison with Nature and not to challenge her. For example, generating electricity is fine, but you should be conscious of how nuclear waste is treated without polluting river water. The same is true for any chemical factory that harms Nature in a larger way. The irony is that America thinks it is happening in the backyards of China or India without realizing its own backyard impacted. Anything you do against Nature anywhere in the World would have its consequences in every part of the World. If you dump food into Ocean directly, it will destroy ecology. We are embarking on a prestigious journey of destroying the ecological balance by rapid urbanization, thus resulting in deforestration.

A thought induced in mind will impact the Nature is a subtle way. You're so delicately made to pick up messages from the Universal consciousness such as using a mobile phone. India or any other country is no better place to live as it blindly follows the United States. So, good part is that universally we are in danger; hence the solution should be universal to all of us in equanimity.

Now, World is talking about the bio-magnetic energy that holds all the objects in the entire Universe. Einstein has proved that every atom is a wave pattern. It aligns to the intuition of Enlightened masters all over the World. In those days where there was no vocabulary to express, these masters had created a cultural transformation by worshipping Nature. This worship had transformed into multitude of forms in India. It basically refers to the workshipping Nature, primarily consists of:

    a.   Land,
    b.   water,
    c.   Fire,
    d.   Air and
    e.   Akash (energy particles).

This is the basic understanding of Hinduism. In ancient India, they worshipped all these five elements and Sun as the primary. In order to teach this theory to young children, they had formulated respective God for each of the above to inculcate good practices of respecting Nature. These five elements of Nature helps human beings in survival in this planet. You'd not survive without any of these five elements in respective proportions. These chemical factories have polluted a few elements and slowly the Ozone layer is also depleting! If it continues then there is a certain destruction possible by Nature as it would try to balance the warm earth with Water. You may want to checkout few videos of Al Gore to realize the perils of global warming. In my view, most of these scientists and politicians are responsible for the above scenario.

The laws of Nature is so precise. If you do not do anything creative, that is fine. I believe being lazy is fine at times, at least you're not over ambitious in the pursuit of destroying Nature in the name of Industrialization. The motive of West rapidly increasing science and technology came from the pursuit of first and second world wars. Today, you're living in a world where is there a 50-50 % probable chances of anyone using it to destroy the planet. Every CEO is only worried about the bottom line profit. What a foolish way? What would he do with all the wealth after diagnosed with Cancer? Cancer is not a disease from external. It is basically your cellular intellegence to rejuvenate itself is lost every 45 days. If it does not get rejuvenated, then it eventually starts dying. This is the result of human's behavior against Nature. It is just the result that you're reaping up based on what you'd sown.

Now, it is not too late to realize the mistake and take corrective actions across the globe to heal thy World. It has to happen from the respective Citizen of the World by peacefully protesting against the respective Corporates and Governments to Stop any act of destruction against Nature. For example, chemical fertilizer companies can transform into organic fertilizers over a period of five years. It is possible to impose by the respective Governments to announce any food poisoning using chemical fertilizers is a criminal act in judiciary.

Infact, you can urge govt. to tranform all animal killings into create a man-made forests by forming a biological diversity. You can convert animal waste into organic fertilizers and it can used for farming. Basically, farming is an art. It can be done with an ecological mindset using organic fertilizer at low cost without relying on chemical fertilizers.

All chemical fertilizers and genetically modifying crops should be stopped completely. Moreso it is possible to ban carbonated drinks, chemical packaged food etc over a period of 5 years. If US starts, rest of the world can be slowly enforced to follow. I see a good trend in India with the ban of usage of plastic covers, however lot needs to be done in terms of conserving forests, laws to protect rapid deforestration. It is possible with each of your support and forums that helps in gainging potential dangers of the World. There is a bigger conundrum in terms of stopping nuclear energy which is a different topic to analyze alternal source of energy.

In my view, the whole of United States is completely Inorganic in the name of science and technology without realizing harmonious ways of living in unison with Nature. Every single product from US is chemical friendly and not human friendly from lipsticks to drinks. The Amercian way of life is the reason for all maladies in life from eating unhealthy food, commercialized chips and flavored water. Moreover the types of alchoholic beverages have lined up creating havoc. You don't need a Phd to demonstrate the harmful effects of drinking and/or smoking. I don't want to state what happens to neurons, then why not the respective Governments ban these products to save millions of innocent consumers?

The US have intelligence to build factories without worrying about polluting the river water. Just watch 'Erin Brocowich' that tells the real story of river water pollution. I loved United States during my stay in the USA between 1997 October till 2002 February. However, didn't realize the background allegations of funding ISS or selling rockets to Pakistan that resulted in 9/11 instance of WTC collapse.

When I lived in USA, I loved seeing people working so hard with the ability to market anything. The government looked absolutely Divine. Alas, after a decade, I realized the real background stories of the US involved with foreign policies and American Imperialism in the name of democracy. Yes, it is democracy at the surface, whilst the real face is clear! With so many citizens of the United States suffering from diseases due to lack of proper food bill to protect the citizens of its own Country. Indeed, it is corporate America, which is responsible for spoiling its own country and the rest of the developing countries like India, China, Pakistan that are following without any common sense. Indeed, India could have investigated the food products imported of chemical fertilizers such as 'Urea' which is killing soil wealth and human existence in this planet. Is this a real freedom?

Is it a real globalization where countries exists without worrying about rest of the World. But Nature has taught a lesson by importing diseases in its own country. US had commercialized everything from food to sex that it suffers from its own maladies. Now, India is helping the country by exporting Yoga. Hope it will not be commercialized. Otherwise, India would follow the footsteps of corporate America. While US has stopped all Nuclear plants, not clear why they're willing to export it to India and other countries for production of electricity. It if had been a good will, perhaps US could train India in alternate source of energy. Can't US find a simple alternative fuel instead of PETROL. There is a bigger politics to benefit the United States that even their countrymen would have no clew about. A common countrymen are not aware as they are extremely busy working. They have been made laborers by the corporate America. Only the greedy politicians and corporate sectors are benefiting by their barbaric activities till-date. They are continuing what Brit's had done a century ago in the name of MNC's.

Perhaps corporate Agriculture is even more dangerous as they would force for mass production using chemical fertilizers. Every government in the World should form consortium to ensure food we eat is safe! The five elements should be declared as common for all and support farmers around the world to produce healthy organic food as per law. It is possible to stop war and pollution. More and more people are taking pledge to support green environment. However, without a larger bill by the parliament, it will not be effective. Hence, I request each of you to stress respective governments to support food protection bills.

You take anything from the USA, it has a greed of politicians in it. Each of these scientists seem to have challenged Nature, hence the result of all maladies. Is it not possible to generate electricity using solar or anything that is eco-friendly. US seem to have implemented in its backyard without worrying about the entire World.

What is the value of all your knowledge so far in science and technology? I wonder if science and technology has helped the citizens of the World to survive peacefully or to live in danger. Today, human beings are the most endangered species in the entire planet and the greedy politicians have killed so many innocent people in the name of war. The vengeance of US war against Japan or any other country has not stopped yet from the days of atom bombing Hiroshima and Nagasakhi. It is still trading weapons to countries such as Pakistan and India.

Indeed, a cold war continues despite your inventions, discoveries into mars and moon. I don't know when it will erupt. sWhat is the value of all inventions and discoveries till date? When people of World are dying out of poverty in Africa, Aisa, Middle East or anywhere in the World. Don't you realize a simple fact that every human being is made of the same mass that was derived from the Nature.

I fail to understand a simple point of what makes United states to feel so proud about. Any of these factors highlighted below makes you feel proud:

a. Colonized the Land of America from the native Americans known as 'Red Indians'…history has it in mass genocide of the American natives - red Indians with reference below:

Reference wikipedia # The "Indian Removal Act" of 1830 attempted to move roughly 50,000 Cherokee, Chickasaw, Choctaw and others from their home to Indian Territory (present day Oklahoma). The U.S. government did not provide any means of transportation, forcing them to walk the 2,200 miles. One can reasonably argue that the U.S. government did fully expect many of them to die on the way — especially children and the elderly. The U.S. government recorded 4,000 deaths on just one of many re-location marches among the Cherokee alone; estimates of the total death toll range from as low as 5,000 to as high as 25,000.

---

    b.   Several civil wars in the USA due to Racial/Ethinic issues till the point Abraham Lincoln (1864), 16th President of the United States passed a bill for stopping slavery for which he had spent his entire life to bring in equality

    c.   Rapid Industrialization causing job losses of many citizens of America

    d.   Major NASDAQ stock market crisis due to lack of regulation resulting many American citizens losing their jobs

    e.   Rapid Offshoring of all non eco-friendly industries to countries like India, China, thus causing pollution in the respective geography.

    f.   Industrialized Agriculture with heavily used chemical fertilizers and genetically modified crops and produce for high yield; thus causing cancer in most of the citizens of America and the World citizens.

g. Veto in the UNO? Without allowing other countries to promote ideas

h. Exporting nuclear wealth to India and Pakistan, thus destabilizing the Asia region

i. Lack of robust governance in foreign policies, resulting in imbalance in the Midde East region.

j. Lack of robust FDA regulated products in carbonated drinks, burger and pizzas etc.

k. Lack of robust policies to govern medical practices such as Allopathy medicines which has many side effects.

l. Lack of robust clinical trials and promoting dangerous drugs as medicines to the citizens of the World and the United States.

m. Lack of holistic treatment for all diseases, resulting in increased diseases such as CANCER. Thus, you've promoted Allopathy

n. Stop conditioning young MINDs with gun culture and help them really thing through harmonious ways of living in sync with Nature.

o. Lack of control over explicit content, violent games in the media regulated by censor board

p. Stop Conducting clinical trials in other countries

q. Trading billions of dollars in war planes, guns used in warfare.

r. Stop investing in DEFENSE, instead allot it to farmer incentives, Organic Agriculture and preservation of forests.

s. Stop plastics all over the World with recycling best practices

How can US authorities, the so called 'land of opportunities' allow companies such as Monsoto. Refer below the toxicologoical dangers of this multi national organization. I heard it is acquired by another multi national, MNC. Shouldn't it be banned for poisoning food at source. It uses glyphosate used as herbicide, which is dangerous to human beings.

*Refer:*https://www.organicconsumers.org/news/monsantos-sealed-documents-reveal-truth-behind-roundups-toxicological-dangers

http://www.seattleorganicrestaurants.com/vegan-whole-food/Monsanto-corruption-gmo.php

These above factors demonstrate the imperialistic nature of the United States. Where is the holistic truth? Each of you're not going to survive beyond 80-100 years as I wish, then why all these politics to amass wealth for individual gains alone. What happened to the greatest king of pop of America, when he tried to change his own nature? I think it is time for the Martin Luther King of America, Abraham Lincoln, Mahatma Gandhi and Vivekananda to arrive with their spirit to create a peaceful revolution against the non eco friendly industries. Because, world is one and the same. You cannot separate land, air, water or fire. All these barriers are man-made, just get rid of it to think as global unit to save the planet and the citizens of the World.

The saddest part is that the politicians of America didn't realize Earth is round. Anything that US has done to export terror to other nations has come back to their backyards as Tornado's and depleted Ozone layer in its own space, which they cannot control as Nature holds it. If you kill so many animals ruthlessly for decorating your own plates, then Nature will showcase her anger in the form of tornado's, wars and floods across the country and world. Because the collective consciousness of these animals will induce environment to act based on the painful sensations. The same is true with the foreign policies that advocate terrorism in other countries. Perhaps, UNO must be empowered to act as an independent body without US's interference. Where is the real democracy if people cannot make real decisions?

What is the value of your entire education system, if you're not able to create a simple realization of equality. The basics of human values are missing in the education system. India had an ancient ways of teaching children which is all gone with the lost cultural heritage by the colonization of British Raj. It is an apathy that India has blindly taken the policies, procedures, judiciary, school, administration system of the British Kingdom. The

Indian school system and culture came to an end
with the lost languages and her heritage with the
barbaric invasions of Mughals since 12th century and
British who had ruled India for over 100 years taking
all the land wealth and gold. Thus, India is trying to
revive her lost glory. The food every children eat in
India contains pesticide, insecticide from the MNC
companies. Urea is primarily consists of Nitrogen
(45%) which kills several microorganisms leading to
depleting soil wealth.

You're divided by color, creed, religion,
language and borders. Who created all of these? Isn't
not the inorganic human mind. Most of the bosses
seems to be ruthlessly pursuing goals of the
Organization at the expense of employees, then how
do you define these Harvard graduates who don't
know the value of compassion? What would be the
measure compassion towards fellow living beings if
the so call educated masses all over the world eat
living beings for food. Isn't that barbaric to kill cattle,
poultry for food with de-forestration. How can these
Phd's are silently consuming non-vegetarian food
with no understanding at all? This is staggering.
There are three primary act due to killing animal for
food:
  a. Killing,
  b. Stealing its body for food,
  c. Taking away its basic freedom of
      survival

You're capable of thinking about it. Your
mind is so intelligent that has been conditioned to

work against Nature. India has been a pioneer in promoting vegetarian food for good health and spiritual progression and living in unison with Nature. Also, since time immemorial India had pioneered the act of maintaining ecological diversity and organic farming. Indeed, India was the first palce which had the heritage of organic agriculture since down the centuries from the Indus valley civilization. Did you know Columbus set out his venture to find India, which was very prosperous in those times and eventually found the land of America!

It's simple truth but profound. What you eat is what you'd become. You may know it, food that you consume everyday becomes juice, blood, fat, bone marrow, bones and sexual vital fluid. Now, the genetic science is pondering over personality traits based on the food that you consume. Have you noticed in most of the Western countries due to harmonal imbalances, young girls achieve puberty much early and the fertility rate of men is also going down. These are the reasons of genetically modified seeds (e.g. BT Brinjal) and challenging Nature due to excessive desires to mass produce everything. It is your science and technology that has caused these maladies. You've had so many inventions and discoveries, has it been used wisely to align with Nature or against Nature. India had most of the Enlighted masters and still has a few those who are promoting vegetarianism all over the World. Did you know the legendary actor and kung fu master. Bruce Lee was a vegatarian? I have seen a Youtube video of

Arnold promoting Vegan, which is a welcome change. You should just allow Nature to do its job!

Anything that arrives in the United States becomes a corporate politics. For example, food, sex, work and rest are all basic needs of every human being. Each of these factoros have been commoditized by the corporate America. For example, All burgers and pizzas which so much of mass production that have chemicals and proved to be very harmful to the human body. It is not requried at all. Why is a simple and natural act of sex is made so much of taboo in the United states? Now, next is medicine. The field of medice has become a joke today with so many health care center's partnering with insurance agents to promote cancer, instead of health and well-being. In the end you'd remain a victim, your children will become victims of Corporate America. It is apparent that the country is not safeguarding the citizens of America. Instead, making money out of each of you. You'd work hard earning income, which eventually becomes an expense at a medical center.

What is the use of it all stressing yourself every day from 9AM-6PM in a day job that has no meaning at all. You should be aware of social, political activites happening aroud you. What is the point in hanging out in bar for a weekend pleasure? It is very enticing but not enterprising in the long term. You're losing your health by all inorganic activities such as inordinate desires in mind as thoughts, actions that loops you into endless cause and effect system where you'd reap up the benefits of actions done (karma) etc. what is the meaning of it in the end. You're being poisoned at one end in the form of inorganic food that you consume, and then you're given medical treatment taking out your hard earned money.

Further, your body has become more disease prone due to lack of realization of self. Otherwise it is not possible to consume alchohol, inordinate sexual desires, smoking cigarettes, eating unhealthy junk food, non-vegetarian etc. Without realizing the basic needs, you've been conditioned to indulge in the name of entertainment. See, what is going to happen to those who'd indulge at an young age. It would result in multiple organ failures and cancer.

The above truths have been hidden from you to make you nump and follow the standards set by the corporates. You've been munching pop-corns in front of TV, resulting in all diseases. I mean, you're constantly conditioned by the hollywood and bollywood anchos who drink and eat organic, whilst you're conditioned to eat everything that is non-sense. Just look at coke and pepsi cans in your garage, perhaps you can make a tower. The chocolates that you've consumed so far, toothpaste that has all inorganic content in it. Now, the respective governments has not created any food protection bills to safeguard citizens of the World. Most of the crops, produce seems to have been either genetically modified or grown with chemical fertilizers.

How many of you know that the food that you consume everyday has slow poison in it? Is it not a staggering truth? You've already destroyed the planet with so much of urbanization resulting in deforestration causing an ecological diaster. At times, I feel most of these scientists have partnered with politicians and businessmen to destroy the planet.

A lot of truths had been hidden by the respective politicians. First they had sold the lands to the greedy corporates. Hence, each of your lands have been abused in the name of fertilizers. For example, usage of 'Urea' had resulted in poisoing food at its roots and lose all its nutritional values. Hence, your cells have lost the ability to regenerate itself. This is called 'Cancer' nothing else. All diseases are man-made and not because of Nature. Nature is ever loving, hence there are few messiahs of the World such as G.Nammalvar, who has contributed to the Organic farming, which is not new, the ancient India had mastered these techniques of creating a bio-diversity.

Today, a lot of companies in the US are trying to claim the copyright. What non-sense, this is a simple ancient wisdom of India and how can anyone claim the copyrights. You should be aware of all the background stories of human beings from mass killings in the name of first and second world war. Now, the much larger threat has come in rapid globalization by industrializing food production. The moment food production is commercialized, there is a larger threat of poisoning at the roots such as usage of chemical fertilizer's.

Did you know how these yummy chicken Nuggets are made. You have enjoyed eating nuggets without even realizing that it was a mass murder. I just saw the crushing machine that sucks chicks in and crushes into pieces. It was so barbaric to even watch. Don't you have kids in your home ? Even if you have slightest intelligence and little aware, you should raise a question and take oath to STOP eating non-vegetarian food. It even saddens me to watch video's of violent killing of animals in slaughter house with yelling cows. Don't you heart to reckon what you're doing? You're consuming it, hence Nature will punish you at some point.

Because you do some programming in a computer, you do not want to realize all these facts. What non-sense is this? If you're not even aware of what you eat, what is the purpose of your survival. You are just another dead being with no sense at all. It is a classic example of how barbaric the corporate World is behaving in a wreckless manner with no concern for living beings. They use a mass murder chopping machine to chop all chicks laid there in the altar drill machine. It is so barbaric. I am sure these actions will yield in negative results to your own children. The same barbaric act is true in ruthlessly slaughtering cattle in the slaughter house. In some countries in the name of religion these poor camels and goats are ruthlessly killed for food in the name of God.

Don't you have any heart at all? Inspite of drinking cow's milk everyday, how can be so barbaric to kill them ruthlessly to taste cow mean, bacon sausage and cheese. Well, drink more alcohol, smoke and enjoy as many women as possible and dine all of the above non-veg that you like the most and see the results in the body in 10-20 years. It is obvious that you're invoking CANCER. Also, remember thoughts contribute to these factors above in aggravating the situation. If you're a non-vegan, be ashamed of your own act. Just throw away all your degree certificates if you have missed a simple point in life.

What is the point in amassing wealth after you're diseased at a young age.A great ancient country along the Indus valley had its unique ways of living in unison with Nature. These siddhars (saints) of India had the profound knowledge of the body, mind and soul. When Maharishi Vethathiri had pronounced these Kundalini techniques around the World, US seems to have ignored it completely, despite his speech at the UNO to stop wars by globalizing borders. He was almost deported from the country, luckily he had narrow a escape out of the country without any major issues for pledging the government towards one governance and stop funding war. This is what happens to every Socrates and christs of the World. Most of the foolish politicians don't understand as they would lose their personal wealth. It is possible if each of you start thinking about it right now to save your children and the World.

My point is that a holistic approach is required to healing body, mind to realize soul underneath the core of mind. You are consuming 1001 products everyday, you should observe each and every aspect from where the crops are grown and how is it processed. For example, sugar whitening process involves chlorination. The same is true with rice polishining to make it look brighter. I realized even fruits and vegetables are polished using wax to make it look fresh. If all packaged food had problems of using chemical preservatives that are harmful in one way from chips, sauce to everything, now we have a different problem with the root of how every crop is using chemical fertilizers that are harmful. Thus, human beings are consuming slow poison resulting in cancer. Almost 30-40% in the US alone has breast cancer in women. I respect each of them and request to protest against the respective governments. Now, some of the BT seeds are being exported from the United States. Now, let us see differences between Organic and Inorganic compounds in laymen terms.

The primary difference between organic compounds and inorganic compounds is that organic compounds always contain carbon while most inorganic compounds do not contain carbon. Also, almost all organic compounds contain carbon-hydrogen or C-H bonds. Note, *containing carbon is not sufficient* for a compound to be considered organic!

Everything is chemical! From sugar that you conume, morning tea, breakfast all. Rice is polished with sulphur. I am not an Agri student, being a computer geek, I feel ashamed of not learning the basics of what I am eating everyday. It's ignorance as you're all busy in doing something for living. This ignorance is not bliss. It is your repsonsibilites to understand and conserve, preserve Nature. What will you do if you have CANCER at an early age. Whatever you have done so far will go waste right. Now, it is time to arise, awake and protest peacefully against the perils of human extinction. India had its ancient pride which is lost because of rapid urbanization. It is apparent with the recent 2016 floods in Chennai metro that all the lakes had transformed in to multistoreyed apartments. What were you doing all the time rather than worrying now. The situation is no different in Bangalore, where I live, the city of lakes had been completely taken up by the likes of large marquee builder. If there is flood like it happened in Chennai will paralize the whole city of Bangalore. But unfortunately farmers within India are not even united, thus fighting for the Cauvery water.

It would have been easier for the Indian government to support farmers by declaring usage of water across India without dams. The flow of water must not be stopped! Nature has designed it so delicate that anything you do with your little brain cannot help in sustainable environment. Look at what you've done so far, all plastics cannot be recycled and manmade. Is there anything in Nature that cannot be recylced. Inorganic is your invention by breaking the carbon molecules with your little intellect. Hence, your insensitivity to everything in the name of science and technology is causing human extinction. Now, mobile towers have made little sparrows almost extinct. Last time when I saw these tiny sparrows, my heart felt joyful as I have seen these little birds in my childhood. After I moved to metro's there were fewer variety of birds. Remember, Einstein said 'when honey bees become extinct, the world would be gone within few months'. It simply implies that the pollination cannot happen. Now, see how much of these chemical fertilizers are killing good insects, good micro organisms and worms in the soil. Hence, this is an ecological disaster and we are harming Nature.

***

Chapter 2

Messiah's of Organic Farming

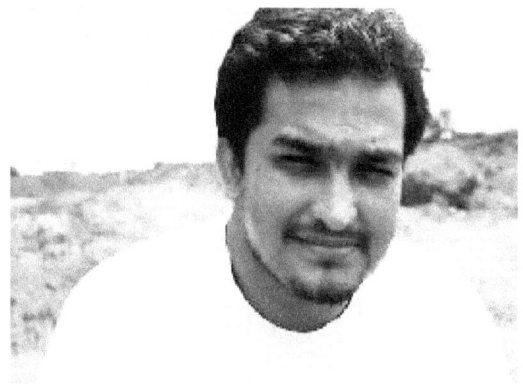

Piyush Manush, *Environmentalist who has created > 100 acre forest on his own in Salem district, TN, India.*

This man is the present and future of India, an environmentalist who has created a forest on his own despite lack of support from the government. Born in Salem, TN, India, he tirelessly working for last couple of decades to save lakes of Salem and further strongly opposed the extraction of bauxite by a major multinational company! Indeed, this had brought him several political wraths both local and international for not allowing multinationals to operate. He has been instrumental in driving several children to understand the values of Nature and help them in conservation. This is a great leadership!

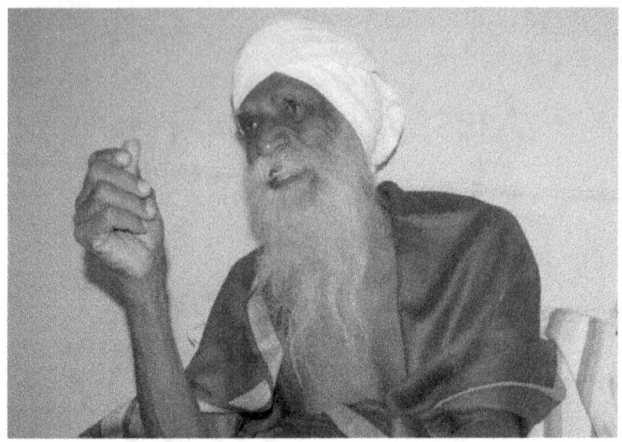

G. Nammalvar, The messiah of Organic farming

Reference # Wikipedia.

G Nammalvar (or **Nammazhwar**) தமிழில்: நம்மாழ்வார் (1938 – 2013) was an Indian organic farming expert, Green Crusader. Hailing from the agro-based Thanjavur district of Tamil Nadu, he was involved in preaching the farmers to get an edge in organic farming.

Nammazhlwar was born in 1938 in Elangadu, Thanjavur District, and he graduated from Annamalai University with a BSc degree in Agriculture. In 1963, he began working for the Agricultural Regional Research Station, a government organization in Kovilpatti, as a scientist, conducting trials on spacing and manure levels of various chemical fertilizers in cotton and millet crops. During his tenure there, the government had conducted various experiments in rain fed land, using expensive inputs like hybrid seeds, chemical fertilizers and chemical pesticides which Nammazhwar considered futile as the rain fed farmers were resource poor. Based on his experience, he felt very strongly that it was imperative to totally reorient the research work being undertaken. But his peers at the institute paid little attention to his advice. Frustrated, he left the institute in 1969.

For the next 10 years, he was an agronomist for Island of Peace, an organization founded by the Nobel Laureate <u>Dominique Pire</u>. His focus was on improving the standard of living through agricultural development in the Kalakad block of Tirunelveli District, Tamil Nadu. It was at this time that he realized that in order to get optimal results in farming, farmers should rely only minimally on external inputs. All inputs should come from within the farm. So called wastes should be recycled and used as input. This revelation was a turning point in his life. He completely lost trust in conventional farming practices and began experimenting with sustainable agricultural methods.

In the late 1970s, Nammazhwar became greatly influenced by Paulo Freire and Vinoba Bhave and their theories on education. The purpose of education should be freedom. Freedom is essentially self-reliance. Self-sufficiency means that one should not depend on others for one's daily bread. Secondly, one should have developed the power to acquire knowledge for oneself. And last but not the least; a man should be able to rule himself, to control his thoughts and feelings.

Eager to propagate these new theories on education, specifically to aid farmers in becoming self-sufficient, he started a Society, Kudumbham in 1979. "Participatory Development" was the way forward. There can be no education without action. Nor can there be any action without education. Both go hand in hand. Nammazhwar interacted with local farmers, understood their needs, and based on their input, evolved farming practices suited to the local farmers.

In 1987, Nammazhwar attended a 4-week training course conducted by the ETC Foundation, Netherlands, on ecological agriculture. In 1990, he founded a network called LEISA (Low External Input and Sustainable Agriculture) to promote the concepts of ecological farming, specifically the importance of self-reliability and low external inputs. During the same year, he started an ecological research Centre for rain-fed cultivation in Pudukkottai district.

Nammazhwar was also greatly influenced by Mr. Bernard de-Clerk of Auroville fame, whom he had worked with since 1984. In 1995 he was nominated as the Tamil Nadu state coordinator for ARISE (Agricultural Renewal in India for Sustainable Environment). Concurrently, Bernard was the coordinator at the national level. During his tenure he travelled widely across India promoting the principles of sustainable agriculture.

When the Tsunami hit India on 26 December 2004, Nammazhwar was actively involved in the rehabilitation process. In 2005, he helped farmers across various villages in Nagapattinam district to rehabilitate. In 2006, he left for Indonesia and assisted in reclaiming several farms in Tsunami affected areas.

Recognizing his extensive work in the field of agriculture, the Gandhi Gram Rural University, Dindugal honored Nammazhwar with a Doctorate of Science degree in 2007.

Nammazhwar travelled widely across the world, observed the agricultural practices in various different ecological systems and based on his findings, trained several farmers and NGO workers. He has written several books and articles in the Tamil language. He had a wide readership across different sections of society. His works may soon be translated to the English language, making his writings easily accessible.

Nammazhwar spent a substantial part of his time actively touring the south and conducting training classes on ecological farming. He was in the process of setting up several researches cum training centers across South India. The first was at Surumanpatti, Kadavur in Karur district. He was also actively involved in linking different farms and institutes around the world so as to accelerate the process of ecological development. [11]

He led the Historic Protest against The Methane Gas project which was started by Great Eastern Energy Corporation an American multinational. The project was proposed in the Fertile Cauvery Delta region of Tamilnadu which is the Source of Food for almost all the people of Tamilnadu. Thanks to his Efforts and the farmer's agitation the project was cancelled.

Nammazhwar was the Chief Guest for the practical session conducted on organic farming titled "iniyellam iyarkai" (Now all natural) on 20-21 July 2013 by the Ramanathapuram district collector.

G.Nammalvars contributions:

At present Indian farming is facing a crisis. More than 0.15 million farmers are forced to commit suicide due to commercial farming that has become economically unviable. Vast stretches of farm land have become saline due to indiscriminate application of chemical fertilizers and pesticides in farming. According to a scientific study, all our food articles are contaminated with pesticides above the limits prescribed by World Health Organization. Citizens are suffering due to pesticide related diseases. Direct benefits of bio-diversity in agriculture lie in the range of eco system services provided by the different bio-diversity components. These include nutrient cycling, pest regulation, pollination and others. (Gunr et all 2003).

The conventional industrial agriculture has resulted in negative consequences affecting ecosystem services and agro ecosystem function. The chemical based monoculture farming system has caused rural unemployment, migration and malnutrition. Children are deprived of childhood and education. To the contrary, organic agriculture benefits from decades of using ecological principles based on diversification and traditional wisdom. It will depend on low external inputs, resources conservation, and biological services. Clearly describe your proposed approach/solution: - 80% of Indian farmers are re-source poor, owning land holding of less than one hectare.

Most of them are less educated. They need demonstration and practical training in natural and material resource management. "In order to fulfill this object, we need learning centers and trainers of both sexes". Organic seeds and cattle breeds are to be collected and conserved. A number of farms are maintained by NGOs and farmers. They need to be up graded more and more youth are to be trained. Suitable learning materials are to be prepared

***

Chapter 3

G. Namalvar's vision!

The ultimate wisdom of Nammal-var's ultimate spirit is echoing in every part of India. May all his visions come true with a lot of youngsters turning into tradition farming techniques in India and guide the world with organic farming.

As discussed, Nammalwar Namalvar is an organic scientist. He was a professor in an agricultural university but he resigned in 1969 and was working in the NGO sector. He has travelled extensively to get people to change to traditional and organic farming. There is a crisis in agriculture in India. Duh! He started by giving some statistics:
- 1/5 Indians are hungry
- 50% children are under nourished

There has been a 12% decline in food consumption from 1990-2001. Around - 2814 children died of malnutrition from Jan-July 2005 in Maharashtra. Malnutrition is hidden hunger, says MS. Swaminathan. About 99% tribal household in Rajasthan, Jharkhand face chronic hunger. Their livelihood is damaged by so-called development activities.

The productivity of land and human beings has been going down.

Around 7.5 lakh hectares of agricultural land is being diverted to non-agricultural purposes every year. Budget allocation to agriculture is only 2%, whereas 65% of population depends on it for their livelihood. Annual spending on irrigation is 0.35%. Wherever suicides are happening in Andhra and Maharashtra, the places are drought-prone. Monsoon rains are predictable. But unpredictable cyclone rains are damaging crops during harvest time. Only 11% of area is under forest cover, come down from 33% a few decades ago. So, no rains!

In summary, there are 2 defects in this model we have adopted - technical & political. After independence, we gave importance to urbanization and industrialization. These rural areas have been completely ignored in the name of urbanization. Agriculture is serving the industries. Did you there had been times of heavy yield recorded during British times. However, we followed America after independence. We imported chemicals. Our own good varieties have been replaced by dwarf varieties that consume more chemicals. Wherever there was green revolution, the soil has become waste. In our culture, the land is treated as goddess. In Western tradition, it is treated as factory. Earth is a place of creation.

In America, there is growing awareness about organic farming, which is acknowledged with pride. However, the real implementation with appropriate bills is still a question. One of the problems with chemicals is water and land pollution. Sir Albert Howard was a British botanist who came to India to teach people Western farming practices but found many farming practices of people very beneficial to the soil, crops, livestock and people (He wrote the book "An Agricultral Testament"). He later said that even the insects were his teachers. There is a right time and place for farming. But, the dwarf varieties are supposed to be poisonous to the insects. Not natural!! These chemical pesticides are called "Aushad", meaning medicine. But it is actually a poison. Didn't you know? Why don't you try some!

Did you know that grapes are dipped in pesticides; from flower to harvest they are dipped 14 times for 14 weeks. The white coating is actually poisoned! It is not fit for eating. Technical difficult is more serious than the political one! In Andhra, 3000 people committed suicide. A retired person from Indian Council for Agriculture wrote a book called "Knowing the Insects". There are 4 stages in the insect life. Eggs, caterpillar, pupa, adult insect - 28 days for a single cycle. Only the caterpillar dies due to pesticides. After 28 days, the cycle continues. The insects have become immune to the chemicals - pesticides immunity.

These pesticides are organo phosphate chemicals. If it enters into our body, it gets deposited in the fatty areas in the brain. It leads to several forms of cancer, hearing disability, loss of memory. Pesticides kill when consumed. But, when we take it indirectly, we get killed slowly. All insects are not our enemies, there are more friends. To eat insects, there are four or five predators. With pesticides, these are also killed. Don't believe my word? Try reading "Friends of Cotton" by two American scientists. The first milk is given by a mother to a child, it contains pesticides. Excessive spraying reaches the land, the grass, the cow, the rivers, cow's milk, into the mother's body. All these are scientific facts, not just activist propaganda. All our agri subsidies are going towards these chemical companies. There are enough predators to protect our crop. Once a farmer sees these, he doesn't know. He panics and sprays pesticides. Also, the predatory birds stop coming after pesticides are applied. With such extensive use of pesticides, the net profit is reduced because the input costs are high.

Instead, all you need to do is to put a chair for the drongo (predatory bird) as a look-out point to look-out for caterpillars! Dragon-flies, wasps are our friends. Even the ones that "Fly like a Butterfly and sting like a bee" like Mohammed Ali. They prey on caterpillars. 75000 tonnes pesticides are thrown around into the environment every year. There is a picture that shows the difference between a fertilized soil and an organically grown soil. The soil that used fertilizers is hard; water runs off it and erodes away the top soil. The soil under organic farming is spongy, with plenty of aeration. This encourages the movement of water and the growth of micro-organisms that release essential minerals for plant growth.

In nature, certain plants like beans and legumes have the ability along with the rhizobium bacteria to do nitrogen fixation that helps produce urea naturally. There are 12000 such plants that could be used as inter-crop or crop rotation. Now, don't even get me started on the problems of fertilizer factories. Okay, you asked for it. I'll just tell you a couple.

Further, the fertilizer factories dig bore wells 1000ft deep and suck all groundwater. The effluents cause huge environmental problems. If you plant a single seedling of paddy, it produces a lot of root and branches. Each paddy grain has capacity to produce 20000 grains. Take a new grain, not more than 15 days old. There should be only a film of water. Flooding the field with water weakens the roots. The all India average yield of rice is 2.5 tonnes/hectare.

In Madagascar, there is space technology deprived Madagascar, gets 21 tonnes/hectare. They use a system called 'System of Rice Intensification' method. Some of the aspects are planting single seedlings, rather than a clump; not flooding the paddy fields. Germany gives $2 per cow as subsidy. Skimmed milk imported here from Germany is sold at the lowest price. Sri Lanka exports coconuts to us. Other countries give export subsidies to promote export to India. Farmers are taking to organic farming in a big way. Even the University of Agriculture is picking up.

The organic fertilizer is called 'Amruthpani', which is made of cow dung, cow urine and jaggery mixture that could be produced within 24 hours is an excellent fertilizer that could be applied topically and also along with the irrigation water. A company called "WR Grace" packaged neem extract. They crushed the neem seeds, and processed it. The extract, when sprayed, is a good fungicide. They have a patent for the extract. This is used extensively in India and in 2000, 5 people from India along with Namalwar fought the case. Neem grows only in India, not growing anywhere. People have known this for a long time. Its uses are common knowledge. 3 criteria have to be present for patent - novelty, invention, industrial application.

In India, we didn't have industrial application - i.e. not packaged neem crushed seeds, not available in low-fat, non-cream varieties with no MSG. Our argument was that they didn't have an invention. Case dismissed! Patent revoked! Same case with turmeric.

Another truth about Genetically Modified foods, farmers, NGOs are resisting. But, politicians, judges are corrupt and all GM seeds have been allowed. Especially, the 'BT'-cotton seeds. Farmer cannot own the seeds. It sounds like a Microsoft licensing agreement. What a pity!

These GM plants produce sterile seeds. So, new seeds have to be purchased every time. Only the mill owner can supply. The shops sell only GM seeds. There is a trap right there. Only field trials are allowed for certain GM crops. The agitation is to destroy the trials. The session ended in some humor and a health tip to drink Panchakavya (a mixture of cow dung, cow urine, curds and jaggery. Apparently, it is distilled too, so it should be ok!) daily!

Nammalvar was very happy to be part of it, and had given a lot of directions and planted a lot of trees, and gave instructions and actually worked with them instead of giving theoretical inputs. He was committed to working here in making a model farm. He was really interested in working with very large number of groups. He communicated in a very simple and straightforward way and easily communicates with all.

G.Nammalvar was one of the very rare people we have in India and we should take care of him. He travels a lot. It would be good if he has the flexibility of resources. He won't be very worried about who supports him or not. Nammalvar thought that the center should become a university (or a learning institute) for everyone including farmers and to their children. At the same time, he wanted to do the same things in other areas. He was conducting training for farmers and felt happy with how it progressed. He had many publications on this work as well.

In India, soil has been contaminated with pesticides. Thus, Nammalvar wanted to immediately stop it by educating farmers to be ecological. Very few people in this country know how to do ecologicaly good farming. These are the times many farmers had committed suicides with little support from the government. Thus, he had a vision of creating model farming best practices with several publications. Throughout India there was a request to develop an organic farming network. Farmers were in isolation. Thus, he ventured in to extensively creating models for sustainable agriculture. Everything needed to be consolidated. With regard to the license to sell organic materials in the market – There is a "participatory gaurantee system" recognized by the IOF and UN. The farmers themselves guaranteed that they are producing Tanjavoor, Coimbatore, Erode etc. -- farmers and consumers formed groups for creating a green shop which is guaranteed organic food.

Nearly 80% of farmers in TN are small farmers under 5 acre land, so they couldn't spend on larger certification. Thus, he certified inspector who could review and certify these farmers. These inspectors didn't have to be any experts. These organic farming best practices spread across Kerala, Andhra, Karnataka, Pondicherry, all are part of this. They were certified to sell all the produce, the millets, rice, the vegetables and fruits, etc.

The suicides came about after the debts became too high. Final solution was to have simple ancient methods in sync with Nature, instead of any costly inputs from the western methods. The only way to solve the food crisis is to have local and ecologically good way -- mixture crops, crop rotations etc. worked efficiently. Primarily rice crops needs a lot of focus. However, there were very less farmers with problems of low-rainfall area where they were working on millets. Hence, G.N involved more in these areas of drought and worked tirelessly towards uplifting these farmers in the region. The food crisis was fueled by cash crop conversion. Every farmer wanted advance cash. So every farm can have a component which can provide the cash part. The ecological farm will have multiple areas with different crops. How easily are folks changing to organic farming -- already some 10000 have been converted, while some 20000 are in the transition stage. Only during the last 5 years farmers are changing over because the crisis is too hard, plus the prices of other commodity is forcing the farmers. If the farmer is committed and well trained, within 3 months he can change over. There are some 20 aspects to this transition. How is the fight against GM seeds? Bio-diversity leads to prosperity. GM seeds are eliminating bio-diversity. Cotton is very prevalent and spreading. But the GM vegetables are being resisted (brinjal, tomato), because of health risks, while cotton is not eatable.

Nammalvar focused on educating the farmers side. What is hard about asking farmers to switch to organic farming – farmers were very worried about economy. The Natural farming is a method which will regulate the cost of the inputs. Whatever you get in the field can be used for farm need and home need. That argument alone works really well. Are the organic products sold at a higher price? -- we have the green shops in many cities (kumbakonam, chennai, trichy etc.). Where-ever we have green shops we sell through it. In the green shop, the wholesale market price goes to the farmer, while 20% goes to the administration of these green shops. So the farmer gets a very good deal on these. Nammal-var is administrator for OFAI which recognizes the participatory guarantee system. Regarding publishing: planning to publish a monthly newsletter in Tamil. It can be printed in English also for the benefit of other states once in 3 months. It would be possible to translate these manuals and booklets -- already they have some requests from Karnataka and Andhra. The different aspects involved in converting a field from chemical fertilizers to organic farming include:

1. vermiculture -- earthworm

2. green manuring -- composting or growing in the soil

3. amrutha paani -- cowdung, cow urine and jaggery. 24 hours tonic is ready and successfully used by farmers.

4. herbal pest repellent -- cow urine based

5. panchagavya -- healthy tonic. Dr. nagara-jan used it on agriculture

6. farmer's cytosum -- coconut milk and but-termilk fermented and diluted with water

7. manure tea -- cowdung, leaves, jaggery, 200 litre drum of water -- 1wk to prepare.

8. gunabasalam -- waste of any dead animal and mix with jaggery and keep for 25 days – 1% solution to be used 9 to 10 eggs in a plastic container and lemon juice is added until eggs are completely submerged. add jaggery and 20 days you have egg-lemon extract.

10. Multiple cropping for greening purpose. maharashtra 4 millet, 4 rice, 4 oilseed, 4 green manure crops -- grow with the above methods.

How to make vermin compost, vermin wash, importance of crop-rotation, mixed-cropping, integrated farming, relay cropping, no tilling farming by choosing coconut, banana etc. are what the farmers are taught in the workshops. Each farmer's field may not need them all. So they follow a method of farm-specific agriculture. The aim is for the farmer to learn what is needed in their field. Minutes of Asha Austin meeting of June 29, regarding Nammalvar's fellowship, and follow-up Q&A in the Asha-Fellows weekly conference call.

Reference:
http://data.ashanet.org/datastore/data/Focusgroups/Fellowships/Proposals/Pending/Nammalvar/

Dr. G. Nammalvar is an organic scientist. He has been working in the area of natural farming for the last 45 years. He was working with government until the Green Revolution came along (and pesticide and chemical use) and since then he has been working with NGO's and other organizations. He primarily worked in Tamil Nadu and in some areas of Karanataka, Kerala, Andhra Pradesh.

He has managed to get 100,000 acres of rice to be grown with natural farming methods. He was part of the team which visited Germany to fight the neem extract patents, and worked on desalinating land after the tsunami . His focus was Organic farming, mixed farming is useful because of the low input costs. A farmer can restore the soil fertility for organic farming within three months by using a twenty point method.

He was trying to make farming viable – that is the fairer way to look at it (how the farmers perceive it). All things along the lines of organic, renewed land, no soil erosion, multiculture, no GM etc. are part of his philosophy, but what the farmers are looking for is low cost. In the context of the current farming crisis low cost is an important solution. Agriculture crisis situation is very serious. He trusted in creation of training & educating materials is very important in the near future. There are approximately 65 ecological centers in TN. He wanted to promote more and want to set up 1000 training centers all over Tamil Nadu in the next 3 years. Also extend to Karnataka and Andhra Pradesh. He planned to work in the low-rainfall areas on TN: Thiruvallur, southern part of Erode and Dindigul and part of Cuddalore.

Let us understand his plans for promoting Integrated Pest Management in Cauvery River Basin (mentioned in Project Proposal). In the Cauvery Delta produces the maximum amount of Rice in TN. -- Even though Rice is the staple food here, farmers were still in debt. The knowledge of Pest Management was very limited here. Hence, there was a need to conduct continuous training programs for the farmers. Dr. G. Nammalvar travelled extensively throughout South India and spent 3 days every month in Trichy and planned to spend time in Cuddalore, where he aspired to set up training center

Dr. had published notes on a) Madagascar method of growing rice - This method produces 2-3 times the yield of rice. b) Biomass and Green-leaf manure.

This is available everywhere, but not used.
c) Amruthapaani
d) Herbal Pest Repellant
e) Panchagavya
f) Vermi-compost
g) Herbal tea preparation.

This works as growth promoter h) egg juice [the concoction with the lime and the fermenting] i) Navadanya - Mixture crop-pattern ensures fixed amount of income j) Mulching - Important organic farming practice used world-over. k) Double-Digging - Improves fertility of soil. l) Azola - Algae used in cattle-breeding and weed-control in paddy fields m) Crop Rotation n) Honey-bee rearing o) Mushroom Cultivation p) Fish culture q) Rain-water Harvesting Q. Who will this material be given to? And published in which languages? -- This material is meant both for trainers and farmers -- Free for farmers, but NGO's can get it for a small fee -- Publish first in Tamil, then English, then in Kannada and Telugu and other languages -- Enough material is already available for these, as he teaches this on a daily basis. Needs to

***

Chapter 4

Epilogue

You can contribute to environment in every possible way from planting a tree, creating forests, growing produce in farm or terrace, educating your children etc. It is even more valuable to educating a farmer about ecological farming by creating a sustainable agriculture without having to buy any fertilizer. Indeed, Dr. G. Nammalvar has planted real green and organic revolution in the hears of younger generation which is growing more and more with his spirit witnessing it in the cosmos.

India has done the ecological farming with the cattle, earthworms, poultry etc. Indeed, it was the greed of rapid industrialization by the western world has caused the havoc. We have poised your body, nature and the world. Today, world is dangerously living with the perils of looming nuclear war, disastrous food produce etc. I pledge to each of you to arise, awake to create awareness amongst farmers. Perhaps, each of you can visit a farm land, adopt or buy and demonstrate the power of ecological farming which can yield better and help you in sustainable farming.

The people of the world should protest peacefully to stop bio-technology seed production known as BT-Brinjal, BT-Potato and stop dangerous science and technology that is turning out to be absolutely destructive. Let us resort to organic ways of living from our self, society and nature.

You must ask question before consuming every meal. Buying

Blessed by the Divine!!!
Blessed by the Divine!!!
Blessed by the Divine!!!

www.ingramcontent.com/pod-product-compliance
Lightning Source LLC
Chambersburg PA
CBHW071329310526
45789CB00017B/2140